CORDYCEPS FOR BEGINNERS

Unlocking Vitality, Harnessing Cordyceps Unveiled For Wellness, Stamina, Healing, Energy, Health, And Immunity

Georgette Lockett

DISCLAIMER

The author of this book is not affiliated, associated, endorsed, sponsored, or approved by any company or individual. The views and opinions expressed in this book are solely those of the author and do not necessarily reflect the official policy or position of any entity.

The author hereby disclaims any relationship, collaboration, or partnership with any company or individual mentioned in this book. Any references to products, services, or individuals are provided for informational purposes only and should not be construed as an endorsement or recommendation.

Readers are advised to exercise their own judgment and discretion when applying the information provided in this book. The author shall not be held responsible for any actions taken by readers based on the content of this book.

This book is intended for general informational purposes only, and the author makes no representations or warranties of any kind, express or implied, about the completeness, accuracy, reliability, suitability, or availability of the information contained herein. Any reliance on the information in this book is at the reader's own risk.

The author reserves the right to update, change, or modify any information in this book without notice. It is the responsibility of the reader to verify any information before taking any actions based on the content of this book.

By reading this book, the reader acknowledges and agrees to the terms of this disclaimer.

Table of Contents

INTRODUCTION

Cordyceps is a fascinating fungus genus with a unique role in traditional medicine, cultural traditions, and modern scientific investigation.

Overview Of Cordyceps

Cordyceps is a kind of fungus that belongs to the Ascomycota family and is found mostly in high-altitude locations such as the Himalayas, Tibetan Plateau, and portions of China.

Cordyceps species are known for their unusual lifestyle, in which they infect and parasitize certain insect larvae before expanding out of the host's body and creating elongated fruiting bodies. This process gives the mushroom-like structure its characteristic look.

Historical And Cultural Significance

Cordyceps has a rich historical and cultural importance since it is strongly anchored in traditional Tibetan and Chinese medicine. It has been utilized in these civilizations for millennia because of its purported therapeutic characteristics and health advantages. In Tibetan medicine, it is known as "yartsa gunbu" or "summer grass, winter worm," while in Chinese medicine, it is known as "Dong Chong Xia Cao," which translates to "winter worm, summer grass."

Importance In Traditional Medicine

Cordyceps has been revered in traditional medicine for its putative adaptogenic, anti-fatigue, and immune-boosting effects. It has been used to treat a variety of health conditions, such as respiratory illnesses, renal abnormalities, and exhaustion, and even to enhance lifespan and vigor.

Modern Research And Scientific Interest

Cordyceps has piqued the scientific community's interest in recent years owing to its possible health-promoting characteristics. To understand its pharmacological effects, researchers have been studying its bioactive substances, including polysaccharides, cordycepin, and different antioxidants. Its potential for boosting immunological function, reducing tiredness, improving exercise performance, controlling blood sugar levels, and even demonstrating anti-inflammatory and antioxidant effects has been studied.

Furthermore, Cordyceps has sparked attention due to its involvement in respiratory health promotion and potential uses in supporting kidney and liver function. Its adaptogenic characteristics, which may help the body adapt to stress, have grabbed the curiosity of both academics and health enthusiasts.

Cordyceps' potential health advantages and processes are being explained as scientific research progresses, adding to its increased appeal as a natural supplement and health-promoting agent in a variety of forms, including extracts, supplements, and teas.

CHAPTER 1

Understanding Cordyceps

Taxonomy And Species Variations

Cordyceps is a genus of parasitic fungus that has received a lot of interest recently because of its unusual life cycle and possible health advantages. Cordyceps taxonomy is varied, with over 400 known species. These fungi are members of the Ascomycota phylum, and Cordyceps is a member of the Cordycipitaceae family within this phylum. Cordyceps militaris, Cordyceps sinensis, and Cordyceps ophioglossoides are some well-known species.

The species of the genus Cordyceps differ in terms of appearance, bioactive chemicals, and ecological habitats. Cordyceps militaris, for example, is often grown for medicinal reasons and differs from the parasitic Cordyceps sinensis, which infects insects and has been used for ages in traditional Chinese medicine.

Habitat And Natural Growth Conditions

Cordyceps fungus have a varied variety of environments, although they are most typically found in mountainous places, including the Himalayas, Tibet, and other parts of Asia. Cordyceps' natural growing circumstances are often defined by precise temperature, humidity, and altitude needs. These mushrooms are most common in chilly, alpine regions.

Cordyceps has an intriguing life cycle in which it parasitizes insects or other arthropods. Fungus spores enter the host organism, and mycelium develops within, ultimately eating the host. The fruiting body, which is the visible component of the fungus, emerges from the host's body.

Lifecycle And Unique Characteristics

Cordyceps' lifespan is tightly linked to that of its host organism. The fungus has developed an entomopathogenic parasitism approach in which it infects and eventually kills insects. The life cycle starts with the distribution of spores in the environment. These spores germinate and infiltrate the host's body when they come into touch with a compatible host.

As the fungus develops inside the host, it passes through many developmental phases before forming the distinctive fruiting body. The emergence of the fruiting body from the host is an eye-catching feature of Cordyceps biology.

Cordyceps has sparked interest not just because of its unusual lifespan, but also because of the medicinal substances it generates. Polysaccharides, nucleosides, and cordycepin are among the substances that contribute to the possible health advantages of Cordyceps supplementation.

Understanding Cordyceps' taxonomy, habitat, lifespan, and distinctive traits offers the groundwork for investigating its diverse uses in traditional medicine as well as current health and wellness activities.

CHAPTER 2

Nutritional Composition Of Cordyceps

Cordyceps is a unique fungus genus noted not only for its unusual lifespan but also for its amazing nutritional content. This chapter examines the numerous nutrients and bioactive chemicals found in Cordyceps, emphasizing its health-promoting qualities and possible human health benefits.

Nutrients And Bioactive Compounds

Cordyceps species are high in several vital nutrients and bioactive substances, which contribute to their nutritional value. The nutritional makeup of Cordyceps varies somewhat across species, but in general, it provides a source of proteins, carbs, fibers, vitamins, and minerals.

1. Cordyceps is a complete protein source since it includes all necessary amino acids. These amino acids are essential for a variety of physiological processes, such as muscular development, immune system function, and neurotransmitter production.

2. Carbs are a main source of energy, and Cordyceps delivers complex carbs that are slowly digested, giving prolonged energy. This might be useful for those who want to keep their blood sugar levels steady.

3. **Fiber:** Cordyceps includes dietary fiber, which aids digestion. Fiber helps maintain regular bowel movements, prevents constipation, and promotes the development of good gut flora.

4. Cordyceps is a natural source of vitamins, including B vitamins (B1, B2, B12, and niacin), vitamin E, and vitamin K. These vitamins are necessary for energy metabolism, immunological function, and general health.

5. **Minerals:** Cordyceps contains essential minerals such as potassium, calcium, magnesium, and phosphorus. These minerals are essential for bone health, muscular function, and the body's many enzymatic activities.

6. **Bioactive substances:** Polysaccharides, nucleosides, and sterols are among the bioactive substances found in Cordyceps. Numerous research have been conducted on these chemicals due to their potential health advantages, which include antioxidant and immunomodulatory capabilities.

Health-Promoting Properties

Cordyceps has a distinct nutritional composition, which adds to its health-promoting qualities. Among the most important factors are:

1. Cordyceps is classed as an adaptogen, which means it may help the body adapt to stress and preserve homeostasis.

This has the potential to improve the management of stress-related diseases and promote overall resilience.

2. **Antioxidant Activity:** Bioactive components in Cordyceps, such as polysaccharides, have antioxidant activity, which aids in the neutralization of free radicals in the body. This antioxidative impact might aid in the reduction of oxidative stress and inflammation.

3. Cordyceps has been examined for its ability to influence the immune system, boosting immunological response and promoting overall immune function. This might be especially advantageous for those wanting to strengthen their immunity.

Potential Benefits For Human Health

The nutritional content and bioactive chemicals in Cordyceps contribute to several potential health advantages, including:

1. Energy and Stamina: Cordyceps has long been used to boost energy and stamina. Athletes and those who lead active lives may benefit from it in terms of endurance and fatigue reduction.

2. Respiratory Health: According to certain research, Cordyceps may have good benefits on respiratory function, making it potentially advantageous for those with respiratory disorders.

3. Cordyceps has anti-inflammatory characteristics that may be useful in controlling inflammatory diseases and improving general joint health.

4. Cordyceps may have a role in controlling blood sugar levels, making it appealing to those with diabetes or those trying to maintain stable glucose levels.

To summarize, Cordyceps is an excellent dietary supplement with the potential to boost general health and well-being due to its nutritional richness and bioactive components. More information on the nutritional advantages and medicinal potential of this intriguing fungus is expected to emerge as a study on it continues.

CHAPTER 3

Traditional Uses Of Cordyceps

Historical Applications In Different Cultures

Tibetan and Chinese Medicine: The most well-known species, Cordyceps sinensis, has long been used in Tibetan and Chinese medicine. It has traditionally been used to boost vigor, stamina, and lung health. It was considered an adaptogen in these traditional medicinal traditions, boosting the body's resistance against adversity.

Ayurveda: Cordyceps (also known as "Keera Jadi" or "Yarsa gumba") has been acknowledged in Ayurvedic medicine for its ability to boost energy levels and support general wellness. It was historically used to treat deficiencies and to boost the immune system.

Folklore And Traditional Remedies

Cordyceps is strongly embedded in Nepalese mythology, where it is known as "Yarsa gumba" or "Yarchagumba." Folktales depict it as a mythological fungus with remarkable abilities, thought to have aphrodisiacal characteristics and to increase strength and lifespan.

Cordyceps has always been kept for the privileged owing to its scarcity and alleged health advantages. It was seen as a prestige and riches symbol and was often worn by emperors and nobility.

Cultural Significance And Rituals

Harvesting Rituals: Cordyceps harvesting is an important occasion in areas where it grows naturally, such as the Himalayan highlands. Harvesters often venture over hazardous terrains during specified seasons to obtain this fungus. Cordyceps is traditionally harvested by carefully extracting it from the soil without harming the host organisms.

Cordyceps' cultural relevance goes beyond its therapeutic properties. It is incorporated into festivals, artwork, and local customs, demonstrating its deep-rooted significance in these places' social and cultural fabric.

Cordyceps, which is profoundly ingrained in many civilizations, has a rich historical importance in addition to its medical usefulness. Its esteemed position, which is entwined with folklore and traditional customs, demonstrates its cultural significance as well as its long-standing relationship with health, energy, and endurance across many communities.

This cultural and historical context enriches its present applications and encourages a deeper awareness of its potential advantages in modern medical and wellness practices.

CHAPTER 4

Modern Applications In Medicine

Research On Medicinal Properties

Cordyceps, a genus of parasitic fungus, has sparked considerable interest owing to the diversity of its bioactive chemicals. A variety of possible health advantages have been discovered via research on its therapeutic characteristics. Immunomodulatory, anti-inflammatory, antioxidant and anti-tumor properties have been studied. Polysaccharides, nucleosides, sterols, and peptides are among the bioactive substances found in the fungus, which contribute to its medicinal potential.

Clinical Trials And Findings

Numerous clinical trials have been conducted to study the health benefits of Cordyceps. These clinical studies cover a wide range of medical concerns, including respiratory illnesses, renal health, cardiovascular health, and immune system support. Trials, for example, have looked at its role in improving respiratory function and exercise performance by increasing oxygen absorption and decreasing tiredness. Cordyceps extracts have also shown promise in the treatment of renal disease and the maintenance of cardiovascular health by controlling cholesterol levels and promoting appropriate blood pressure.

Cordyceps In Pharmaceuticals And Supplements

Cordyceps' therapeutic characteristics have led to its use in medications and nutritional supplements. Cordyceps extracts and formulations are available in a variety of forms, including capsules, powders, and tinctures. These items are often sold for immune support, vitality, and general well-being.

Cordyceps-based medications are being investigated by pharmaceutical firms for their potential use in treating a variety of illnesses. Cordycepin, a molecule found in Cordyceps, has been shown in laboratory research to have antiviral characteristics, sparking interest in its potential usage in antiviral treatments.

Despite the encouraging results, it is important to stress that additional extensive clinical trials and long-term investigations are required to properly confirm these medical uses. Standardization of extraction processes and dosing procedures is also critical for guaranteeing the effectiveness and safety of Cordyceps-based medications and supplements.

Understanding Cordyceps' present medicinal uses provides a look into its potential benefits to healthcare, but more study is required to fully exploit its therapeutic qualities.

CHAPTER 5

Cultivation And Harvesting

Cordyceps, an enthralling fungus genus, has long been renowned for its therapeutic powers. Traditional harvesting techniques, which mostly included natural gathering, were fairly restricted owing to the scarcity and seasonal availability of wild Cordyceps species. However, as demand has increased and cultivation techniques have advanced, more sustainable and regulated approaches have arisen.

Cultivation Methods

Substrate-Based Cultivation: Growing Cordyceps on a substrate is one of the most common ways. Grains infused with the fungus mycelium, such as rice, oats, or sorghum, are common substrates. This approach enables regulated development in a controlled environment, simulating the natural growth circumstances.

Liquid Fermentation: Another method is liquid fermentation, in which mycelium is grown in liquid media. This approach often improves active ingredient bioavailability and enables large-scale synthesis in bioreactors.

Harvesting Techniques

Harvesting mycelium entails carefully removing the mycelium or fruiting body of the Cordyceps. Harvesting processes may differ depending on the species and the precise section of the fungus utilized for therapeutic reasons.

Precision and timing: Harvesting time is critical since it impacts the potency of the active chemicals. For example, collecting Cordyceps at the appropriate time of development provides the optimum concentration of bioactive chemicals.

Challenges And Advancements In Large-Scale Production

Quality Control: It is vital to maintain quality standards in agriculture. Controlling parameters like as temperature, humidity, and sterility during the growing process is critical for maintaining the end product's potency and effectiveness.

Given the fungus's historical scarcity, sustainable production techniques are critical to preserving both the fungus and its ecology. Researchers and farmers are always looking for new methods to reconcile rising demand with environmental concerns.

Technological improvements: In recent years, technological breakthroughs have changed Cordyceps farming. To optimize growing conditions and increase yield, bioreactor systems, genetic engineering, and new substrates have been developed.

Market Difficulties: While cultivation has expanded Cordyceps availability, assuring authenticity and quality in the market remains a concern. Some goods may claim to include Cordyceps, however, they may be contaminated or of poor quality.

Cordyceps cultivation and harvesting have seen considerable changes, transitioning from conventional wild gathering to controlled, sustainable growing techniques. These developments not only boost availability but also allow for improved quality control and possibly more cost-effective manufacturing, all of which contribute to its larger accessibility and prospective uses in a variety of sectors, including medicines and functional foods.

CHAPTER 6

Cordyceps In Sports And Fitness

Performance Enhancement Properties

Cordyceps is thought to provide potential benefits for athletes and fitness enthusiasts. Its active components, including cordycepin, adenosine, and polysaccharides, are said to promote physical performance by improving oxygen use, increasing ATP synthesis, and optimizing energy metabolism.

1. **Increasing Oxygen Utilization:** Cordyceps is thought to promote cell oxygen intake. Enhanced oxygen consumption may help in the transport of oxygen to muscles, thereby postponing exhaustion and enhancing overall performance during severe physical exercises.

2. **Energy Production:** The basic energy carrier in cells is ATP (adenosine triphosphate).

Cordyceps chemicals are thought to boost ATP generation, giving a more sustainable energy source throughout exercises, which might translate to better endurance and less tiredness.

3. Cordyceps is classified as an adaptogen because it helps the body cope with stress. This adaptogenic characteristic may benefit athletes in dealing with physical stresses, promoting faster post-exercise recovery, and lowering the risk of overtraining-related disorders.

Athletes' Use And Impact On Endurance

Athletes from a variety of sports have investigated Cordyceps pills or extracts to see whether they might improve their physical performance. Long-distance runners, bikers, and mountaineers, in particular, have shown interest because of the purported gains in stamina and oxygen usage.

According to research, Cordyceps supplements may improve endurance levels. Some people have shown gains in aerobic capacity, exercise performance, and fatigue reduction in studies. The level of its effects, however, may vary across people and may not generate the same outcomes for everyone.

Ethical And Regulatory Considerations

Regardless of the possible advantages, using Cordyceps or any other supplement in sports involves ethical and regulatory difficulties. Certain medications or supplements that may boost performance beyond natural capabilities are restricted or banned by several sports organizations and regulatory bodies. While considered a natural chemical, cordyceps may come under investigation in competitive sports owing to its alleged performance-enhancing properties.

To achieve compliance with anti-doping procedures, athletes must be informed of the rules and regulations governing supplement use in their particular sports. While Cordyceps is generally thought to be safe, checking purity and quality when purchasing supplements is critical, since impurities or adulteration may result in unwanted effects or disqualification in sports contests.

To summarize, although Cordyceps shows promise in improving physical performance and endurance, its influence varies depending on the person, and its use in sports needs careful evaluation of ethical, regulatory, and possible health consequences.

CHAPTER 7

Cordyceps In Traditional Chinese Medicine

TCM Principles And Cordyceps

Cordyceps, also known as "Dong Chong Xia Cao," is adored in TCM for its alleged capacity to tonify the kidneys and lungs. It is said to have warming effects and is related to the kidney and lung meridians. The kidneys, according to TCM philosophy, play an important role in managing general health, vitality, and aging, while the lungs manage breathing and the immune system. Cordyceps is often utilized to balance and support these organs, supporting general health.

Prescriptions And Formulations

Cordyceps is often given in different formulations in TCM. It may be used alone or in combination with other plants and chemicals to generate tailored prescriptions. These formulas may differ depending on the exact condition being treated and the patient's constitution. To increase its medicinal properties, it is often mixed with herbs such as Ginseng, Astragalus, or other tonics. Cordyceps is used by TCM practitioners to treat kidney-related illnesses such as exhaustion, weakness, poor libido, and respiratory difficulties such as asthma or persistent cough.

Integrative Medicine Approaches

Cordyceps has received attention outside of conventional methods because of the rising interest in integrative medicine. Integrative medicine blends traditional Western medicine with alternative medicines such as Cordyceps. Because of its potential health advantages, researchers and healthcare practitioners are looking at methods to include Cordyceps in contemporary treatment procedures, particularly in areas such as immune system support, stamina improvement, and respiratory health.

Cordyceps' adaptogenic characteristics have sparked attention in integrative medicine, notably in stress management, sports performance enhancement, and general vitality support. It is often used alongside conventional therapies as part of this strategy to supplement their benefits and enhance overall well-being.

Understanding how Cordyceps fits within TCM provides insight into its historical usage, cultural relevance, and role in current integrative medicine, demonstrating the flexibility and plasticity of this interesting fungus within many healthcare systems.

CHAPTER 8

Ecological Importance Of Cordyceps

Cordyceps, a unique fungus genus, plays an important ecological function in a variety of environments, acting as both a parasite and a helpful organism. Understanding its ecological significance entails investigating its relationships, influence on ecosystems, and conservation and sustainability activities.

Role In Ecosystems

1. Cordyceps has an intriguing life cycle due to its parasitic nature. Certain Cordyceps species parasitize insects, mainly targeting caterpillar larvae. Cordyceps spores infect the insect and germinate, populating the host's body and modifying its behavior. The fungus then multiplies inside the animal, ultimately killing it.

2. Insect Population Regulation: This parasitic association helps to regulate insect populations in a variety of habitats. Cordyceps mushrooms may avoid an overpopulation of insects by limiting their populations, which may have an indirect influence on other flora and animals in the environment.

3. Cordyceps continues to develop after the infected insect dies, eating host tissues and assisting in the breakdown and recycling of nutrients. This mechanism helps with nutrient cycling in the soil, which benefits other creatures and the health of the environment.

Interactions With Other Organisms

1. Some Cordyceps species have symbiotic interactions with other creatures, such as plants. These fungi form mycorrhizal connections with plants, increasing nutrient intake and delivering useful chemicals.

2. Biodiversity Support: The presence of Cordyceps is often associated with a healthy and diversified ecology. They contribute to the overall biodiversity and functioning of these settings as part of the intricate web of interactions within ecosystems.

Conservation Efforts And Sustainability

1.   Overharvesting   and   Overexploitation: Overharvesting poses a concern to Cordyceps species, particularly those employed in traditional medicine. Overexploitation may cause ecological imbalances and the extinction of specific species, affecting both the fungus and the habitats in which they live.

2. Conservation Measures: Conservation efforts are undertaken to preserve Cordyceps species via sustainable harvesting techniques, culture methods, and habitat conservation. Sustainable harvesting includes rules that avoid overharvesting and encourage responsible methods.

3. Scientific study focuses on understanding Cordyceps life cycles, environmental needs, and interactions throughout ecosystems. This understanding contributes to the development of conservation strategies that protect this fungus while preserving the ecological balance.

The ecological relevance of Cordyceps goes beyond its therapeutic and commercial worth, highlighting the need to keep these mushrooms within their native ecosystems for the general health and sustainability of varied environments. Conservation and sustainable practices are critical to preserving this fragile ecological equilibrium.

CHAPTER 9

Potential Side Effects And Risks

While cordyceps is renowned for its potential health advantages, it may have certain side effects and related concerns.

Safety Considerations

1. **Allergies and Sensitivities:** Cordyceps supplementation or intake may cause allergic responses in certain people. Fungi or mushroom allergies may raise the likelihood of harmful responses.

2. **Quality and Purity:** Buy Cordyceps from reliable suppliers to prevent contamination or adulteration, which may result in unpleasant side effects. Product authenticity and quality are critical for safety.

Possible Adverse Effects

1. When using Cordyceps pills, some people may develop digestive disorders such as stomach pain, diarrhea, or nausea.

2. **Drug Interactions:** Cordyceps may interact with certain medicines or substances. It's a good idea to talk to a doctor, particularly if you're on medicine for a chronic ailment or going through treatment.

3. Cordyceps has the potential to have modest blood-thinning characteristics. Individuals using blood thinners or suffering from bleeding problems should take care and seek medical guidance.

Contraindications And Precautions

1. **Pregnancy and Breastfeeding:** There has been little research on the safety of Cordyceps during pregnancy and breastfeeding. To be on the safe side, it's often advised that pregnant or breastfeeding women avoid taking Cordyceps supplements.

2. Autoimmune Disorders: People with autoimmune diseases should consult with their doctors before taking Cordyceps, as it may modulate the immune system.

3. Surgery and Bleeding Disorders: Due to the potential blood-thinning effects of Cordyceps, individuals undergoing surgery or suffering from bleeding disorders should inform their healthcare providers about their use to avoid complications.

While Cordyceps is generally regarded as safe for most people when taken in appropriate doses, it is critical to be aware of potential risks, particularly for certain populations or when combined with specific medications or conditions. It is best to consult a healthcare professional before beginning any new supplement regimen to ensure safety and minimize potential side effects.

Always prioritize quality products from reputable sources, and follow professional advice for personalized Cordyceps supplementation recommendations.

CHAPTER 10

Future Prospects And Research Directions

Emerging Trends In Cordyceps Research

Because of its diverse bioactive compounds and potential health benefits, cordyceps has become an increasingly important focus of scientific research. Interdisciplinary studies examining its pharmacological, nutraceutical, and biotechnological applications are emerging trends in Cordyceps research. Analytical techniques, genomics, and metabolomics advances are revealing new bioactive compounds and elucidating their mechanisms of action. Understanding Cordyceps at the molecular level is becoming increasingly important to effectively harness its therapeutic potential.

Untapped Potential And Unexplored Applications

The vast biodiversity within Cordyceps species suggests untapped potential for discovering new bioactive compounds and health benefits. Exploring lesser-known species or unexplored habitats may lead to the discovery of novel chemical constituents with promising applications in medicine, agriculture, or biotechnology. Furthermore, investigating synergistic effects with other natural substances or medications may lead to the discovery of new therapeutic avenues.

Areas For Further Scientific Investigation

1. **Molecular Mechanisms:** It is critical to gain a better understanding of the molecular mechanisms underlying Cordyceps' therapeutic effects. This includes investigating interactions with cellular

pathways, gene expression, and signaling cascades to fully understand its mechanisms of action.

2. Clinical Trials and Efficacy: We are conducting rigorous clinical trials to validate Cordyceps' efficacy in a variety of health conditions, such as immune modulation, anti-inflammatory properties, and effects on metabolic disorders.

3. Bioavailability and formulations: Improving active compound bioavailability and developing novel formulations or delivery systems to improve absorption and efficacy.

4. Understanding the ecological role of Cordyceps, its interactions within ecosystems, and the impact of environmental changes on its growth and proliferation.

5. Standardization and safety: Thorough evaluation of safety profiles, potential side effects, and establishment of standardized quality control measures for Cordyceps products.

Conclusion

Recap Of Key Points

Throughout this investigation, Cordyceps has emerged as a unique organism with historical, medicinal, and ecological significance. Its taxonomy, lifecycle, and nutritional composition have all played important roles in understanding its wide range of applications across cultures and fields.

Cordyceps is more than just a medicinal fungus; it is an integral part of various cultures, offering remedies steeped in tradition. Its nutritional profile and bioactive compounds have demonstrated enormous potential for health promotion, ranging from immune support to potential therapeutic applications in modern medicine.

Closing Thoughts on its Future and Potential Impact: The journey through the facets of

Cordyceps reveals promising prospects. Modern research is constantly uncovering new health benefits, demonstrating its potential in combating a variety of health conditions. Its inclusion in pharmaceuticals, supplements, and even traditional medicine attests to its importance.

Cordyceps' ecological role as an ecosystem regulator highlights the importance of preserving its habitat. Sustainability efforts are critical for preserving biodiversity and ensuring the survival of this organism.

In essence, Cordyceps crosses boundaries, bridging ancient wisdom with modern science, and holds the promise of significantly contributing to human well-being while emphasizing the importance of conservation.

As we embrace Cordyceps' significance, its story continues to unfold, offering hope, possibilities, and a fascinating journey that intertwines tradition, science, and the delicate balance of nature.

As Cordyceps continues to captivate scientific interest, interdisciplinary collaboration among botanists, mycologists, pharmacologists, and biotechnologists will be pivotal. This collaboration will drive innovative research, paving the way for novel therapeutic applications and sustainable utilization of Cordyceps resources. With a holistic approach encompassing traditional knowledge, modern science, and technological advancements, the future holds promising prospects for Cordyceps in various fields, from medicine to ecology and beyond.

THE END

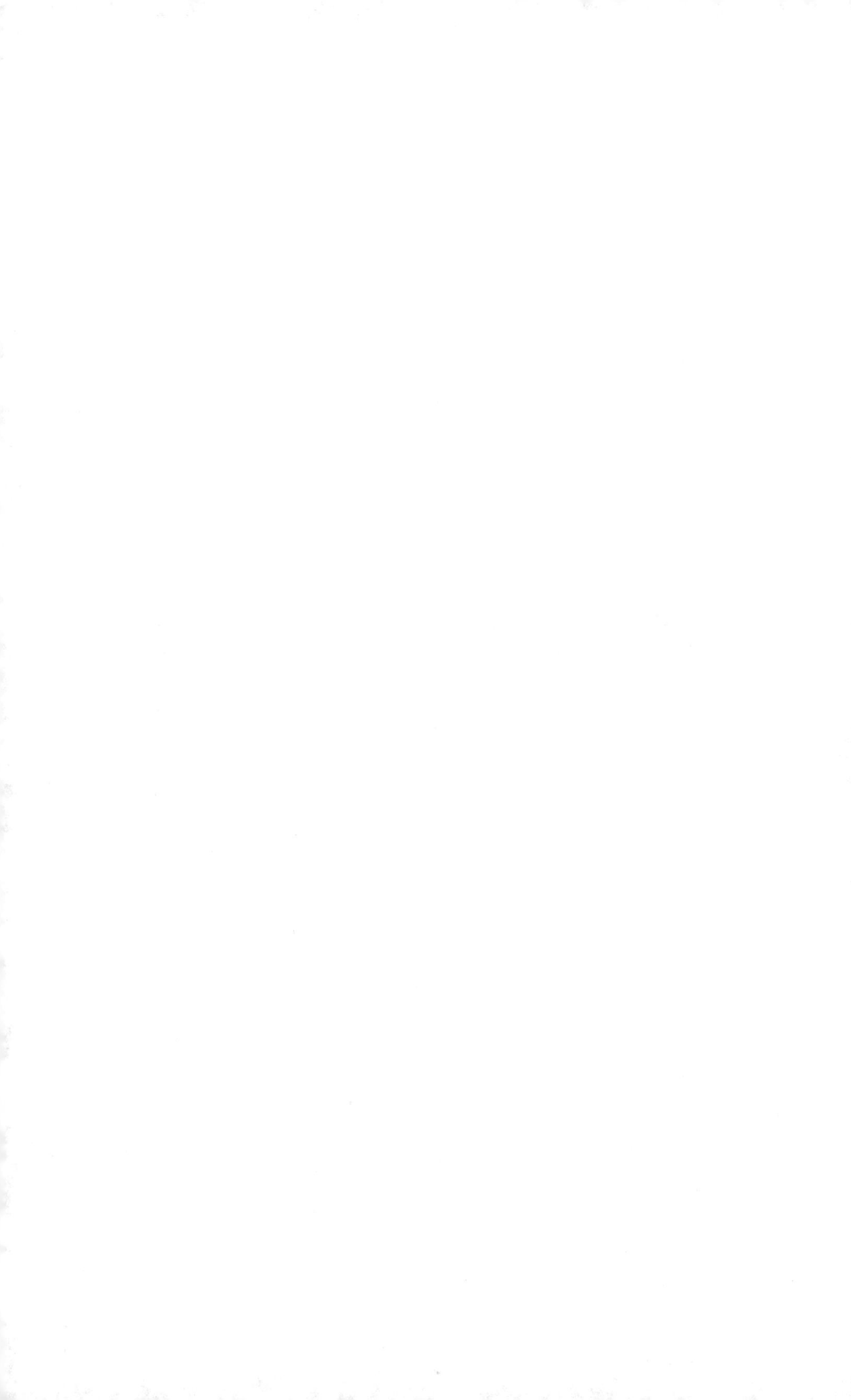